Let Discomfort Be Your Guide

HOW TO UNDERSTAND WHAT YOUR BODY IS TELLING YOU

TERRY DREW KARANEN

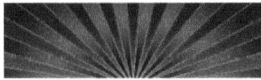

TEIWAZ PUBLISHING

a TDKM, LLC company

Carlisle, Pennsylvania, U.S.A

Let Discomfort Be Your Guide:
How to understand what your body is telling you

by Terry Drew Karanen

Published by: Teiwaz Publishing, Carlisle, Pennsylvania, USA

Teiwaz Publishing is an imprint of TDKM, LLC

TerryDrewKaranen.com

Printed in the United States of America
First Published December 2020

Karanen, Terry Drew

Let Discomfort Be Your Guide: How to understand what your body is telling you / by Terry Drew Karanen

Discomfort is a natural reaction that, while uncomfortable, can hold many answers for us. Is the discomfort telling us to stop, or is it an indication we should push through to a new level in our lives? Whether to stop or push through is discussed in light of all five areas of life: Health, Wealth, Love, Career, and Spirituality. Writing exercises are included to help the reader process thoughts and concerns that may arise.

ISBN: 978-1-893268-11-1 (paperback)

ISBN: 978-1-893268-12-8 (eBk)

ISBN: 978-1-893268-13-5 (PDF)

Printed in the United States of America

Let Discomfort Be Your Guide

Contents

Background

I have lived with many types of pain in my life, both from a physical and mental health standpoint. I suffered with the pain of migraines until I found a doctor and procedure in 2017 that changed my life. Today I am nearly migraine-free. Migraines taught me how to live with both physical and mental pain, which wasn't a healthy way of life. I existed for many years buying into the idea there was nothing I could do to change my condition or life course in general.

In May of 2018, Dr. Ronald G. Barsanti, MD, performed surgery on me to repair a right, inguinal hernia. Dr. Barsanti is a general surgeon practicing in the Harrisburg, Pennsylvania, area, and board certified by the American Board of Surgery. He was educated at the Medical College of Virginia and performed his residency at Penn State Milton S. Hershey Center. Dr. Barsanti is highly respected in the community, and more importantly to me, was personally recommended by my nurse practitioner.

Some months after my hernia surgery, I was still having aching and sometimes stabbing pain at or near the incision. Follow-up visits with Dr. Barsanti indicated my body showed every indication of healing. I was told to gradually begin returning to my normal activities, which meant resuming activities such as carrying mulch around the yard, moving heavy carts in my work life, and weightlifting.

I was genuinely concerned I would do too much and could somehow damage the repair work Dr. Barsanti had done. "How do I know how much I can do?" I asked. Dr. Barsanti told me to take it easy at first and gradually work up to getting back to my normal levels of physical exertion. *Take it easy at first?* Exactly what did that mean? How would I know what was too much? What limits should I put on myself?

I was sitting on the examination table looking for direction from Dr. Barsanti, who was leaning against the counter across from me. He smiled, as he frequently does. That is a beautiful quality in a caregiver. He was never cavalier nor made me feel my concerns were invalid or ill-advised. He wasn't interested in telling me what to do specifically or how I should be doing it. Instead, he listened attentively to the concerns I had about my recovery with earnest concern.

Dr. Barsanti then said five simple words in answer to my question. What he said was,

Let discomfort be your guide.

I thought about those words for the rest of the day. I wasn't given a list of dos and don'ts. I was assured the surgery had been a success. I couldn't do anything to cause a relapse *if* I let discomfort be my guide. My surgeon put *me* in charge of my recovery. He trusted *me* to know what was best for my own body.

The approach of working with the patient instead of dictating everything the patient should and shouldn't do is a new model of western healthcare. Working together toward a healing, instead of using a traditional top-down approach, provides the patient with autonomy. Studies have indicated more autonomous patients exhibit increased longevity, while reporting lower levels of stress and less pain (Personal interview, Mausteller, 2020).

You and I live in a time when it's more common for patients to work with their health practitioners instead of following orders from them. It isn't the way most of us were raised. Parents make various decisions for children (rightly so in many cases) of what's right and what's wrong. Religion and our school systems put restrictions on children that, while perhaps well-meaning and arguably necessary at times, do little to encourage youngsters to explore who they are as unique individuals.

This upbringing, along with societal expectations of what should and shouldn't be done, continues to affect the way we make choices in our lives as we mature into adulthood. Being in charge of one's life can be an unsettling situation if we are used to being told what to do and when.

Over the following weeks I found my body didn't always respond the way I thought it should when applying the advice given to me by Dr. Barsanti. I took note of what worked and what didn't. I also discovered a duality in the presence of discomfort. Sometimes the discomfort seemed to be telling me to back off.

Other times, however, it seemed as though my body was advising me to push through. Duality can be difficult concept to accept for people who want a rock solid, unchangeable either/or, yes/no, or do/don't rule to follow. I began to wonder what was causing the differences in my own life.

The conflicting responses I received from my body helped put me back on a path of healing from the surgery and in other areas of my life. Discomfort of any kind, in particular discomfort accompanied by pain, can be all-consuming. My spiritual beliefs are the foundation of why I take personal responsibility for the life decisions I make each day. The pain I was having from my recovery had led to a crisis of faith. It wasn't in the ability of my surgeon. It was the difficulty of believing in my ability to affect a healing. This book tells that story, which I hope will assist you in learning how to use the discomforts in your own life to your advantage.

Chapter One

What is Discomfort?

Have you experienced discomfort in your life? It would be surprising if you hadn't at some point. There are various types of physical discomfort including:

- Pain
- Aches
- Soreness
- Tenderness
- Irritation

Discomfort also shows up in the areas of our mental health and emotions, often with physical manifestations. Some of these include:

- Nervousness and sweaty palms
- Fear and shaking of our body or extremities
- Anger and a rise in blood pressure

- Sadness and the expression on our face
- Depression and the way we carry our body
- Anxiety and how it can make our heart race

Can you relate to any of those physical or emotional experiences? I can and probably so can you. As humans you and I have numerous ways to define our mood and physical well-being throughout the day. The question is, What do we do with the information?

Few people would seek out discomfort. The American pharmaceutical industry is banking on just the opposite. Traditional western medicine frequently includes a pain reliver, or discomfort reliever, regardless of the situation. While pharmaceuticals help us live better lives every day, the possibility of their misuse is all too clear in our society today.

The U.S. Department of Health and Human Services (HHS) has deemed the misuse of medication so important there is within the HHS a sub-agency, the Substance Abuse and Mental Health Services Administration (SAMHSA). And, within SAMHSA, the Center for Behavioral Health Statistics and Quality (CBHSQ) is the leading federal agency for behavioral health data and research.

Various data collection methods are used to compile this information. This includes national surveys, the behavioral health treatment system, and the national registry for evidence-based programs and practices. In other words, this use of pharmaceutical medication is an excessively big deal in our society.

This isn't, however, a book about the dangers or ill-advised schemes of Big Pharma. It's often true that holistic methods of relieving discomfort can be just as effective for certain situations as their lab-created chemical compound counterparts. While both have their place to help people live better lives, they also share a common dilemma. Are we masking pain or discomfort temporarily, or as a way of life? Do we take a drug or a homeopathic remedy to stop the symptoms, so we don't have to address the cause?

In the United States of America, we have a *disease maintenance system,* not a healthcare system. When we find something physically or psychologically out of balance modern medicine and ancient healing modalities both have protocols as to the course of action our practitioners should recommend. Even if those methods differ or are at times diametrically opposed to one another, they have at least one thing in common. They are all provided to us with the hope or faith that what we take or do will relieve us of the symptom.

That's fine for the moment. The headache goes away and we enjoy the rest of our day. What happens when the headache returns tomorrow, and the next day, and so on? There has to be a reason for the discomfort, a root cause of our pain and suffering. The choice remaining for you and me is whether we want to alleviate the problem and be comfortable for the time being; or, if we want to address the problem(s) or the reason(s) we are having the pain in the first place so we can find a more permanent solution.

The first path is the most common one in our society. There are times when we just want the pain, the soreness, or the headache to go away. The second path requires a greater amount of effort on our part, which may include lifestyle changes we might not be willing to implement immediately. This book does not seek to make either choice right or wrong. It suggests techniques to be more involved in our healing as opposed to remembering where the painkillers are in our medicine cabinets.

Chapter Two

How Does Discomfort Show Up?

Discomfort, pain, anxiety, or an over-all feeling of uneasiness can show up in our lives in numerous ways. The triggers are unique to each of us. A flat tire to one person may feel like the last straw in a string of recent events. To another individual it might be a minor inconvenience, allowing time to read the last chapter of a great book while waiting for AAA® to show up and change the tire.

There are some major changes in our lives which can be the source of our discomfort. These are universal in nature. They include the death of a spouse, child, or other significant person in our lives; moving our residence; starting a new job; finishing a project, such as graduation from college or university; or, getting married or divorced.

You might be wondering how some of those examples could possibly create discomfort. Getting the new job we have been striving to obtain for years or completing our doctoral degree might not seem to be an uncomfortable situation, yet they can be. Why? Because they involve change.

How we react individually to change may also carry over into our society in general. The 2020 COVID-19 pandemic, referred to by some as, "The Great Pause," exacerbated a wide variety of existing situations. Cases of depression, anxiety, chronic illness, anger, and domestic violence began to spike by the beginning of 2020 (Kofman & Garfin, 2020).

Change and New Opportunities

As human beings we find comfort in sameness because we believe it provides consistency in our lives. You or I may have taken the same route to work for over a decade; a new job can cause us to drive in the opposite direction. There are new traffic patterns and time factors about our commute we no longer have down pat. Or perhaps we realize our favorite place to stop for coffee is no longer on our drive.

Even happy events signal the end of something, a loss of some kind. We might think finishing any degree would be cause to feel overjoyed. Of course, this feeling exists, as well it should.

However, we're also giving up part of our identity, that of a student. We're excited about getting into our chosen career field and using the skills we've obtained. It might also include a dramatic change in our lifestyle, both for ourselves and our family. We're suddenly more available thanks to less time needed to attend classes, study, and write papers. For the past four, six, or more years we've lamented about all the things we couldn't do because of our education requirements. Once we have the time to breathe, we could find ourselves feeling a bit lost and confused about what to do next.

The solution is one of those life situations in which we find a paradox: The answer is simple, yet the action we must take may not be easy. Part of the reason you and I have this dilemma is the stories we tell. We believe our stories are the truth. Quite often they're not.

What is a *story*? A story is the tale we tell of why we cannot do what it is we say we want to do. In some cases, it can be the memory of what we believe to be the reason, person, or circumstance that caused a failure of some kind in our lives. In severe situations, it can be what a person has used for years to stay securely in the identity of a martyr or victim.

One disturbing case in my practice involved a woman in her mid-40s who maintained she couldn't hold down a job, or even sit still for more than a few minutes. She told everyone this was due to an instance of child abuse by her uncle when she was only four years old. Her story had been told and retold for most of her adolescent and adult life to anyone who would listen, though she admitted she'd never sought professional help.

Another client was a man who lamented he couldn't hold down a job, didn't have a decent place to live, and longed for a relationship. In listening to his story, he mentioned addiction issues. To deal with those problems he attended no fewer than seven 12-step meetings per week for a number of years – for seven different kinds of addictions, including alcohol, smoking, heroin, overeating, and gambling. I'm careful to say he "attended" meetings. When asked about his sponsor in any of these programs or on which step in the program he was working he confessed he didn't have a sponsor, nor had he begun working his program(s).

Both of these cases are tragic, though not uncommon. They aren't shared with the intent of minimizing the horror of child abuse or addictions of any kind. They are examples of how a story or stories of events in our lives can become the basis for our present circumstance or future outcomes. There's also another way we can use stories: To avoid uncomfortable social situations.

My Grandma Esther frequently used rheumatism and arthritis to avoid social engagements she had no inclination to attend. It never occurred to her to say, "Thank you for asking. No thanks." She felt she needed an excuse not to go somewhere she might have been expected to go. It was easier for her to say, "I just can't, honey. My rheumatiz is actin' up again and you know how that is. I wish I could." This shows how our excuses can also be our stories (Karanen, 2018).

Stories are usually not factual, though the situations which make up the story are. They become a convenient excuse to avoid uncomfortable situations. Without them we might have to stretch a little outside our comfort zone, which immediately triggers a discomfort response. Stories can also be a way to manipulate people. Grandma's excuse got her out of going to some party with people she didn't care for. It also garnered her a rather large dose of sympathy. "Oh, poor Esther," was not an uncommon phrase when she was being discussed by others. She was receiving attention and concern from others, which she craved, although the mechanism she used to achieve the result was emotionally unhealthy.

Where can you and I turn when we experience discomfort in some area of our lives? How can we know if the choices we make are buying into a story, one keeping us stuck where we are, or signaling an indication we're ripe for change to create the life we want to live?

Divine Guidance or Intuition?

If we let discomfort be our guide, then we're opening ourselves up to taking charge of our lives. We must "look within" to find our answers. In other words, we're faced with the decision of which path to take at the fork in the road: Stop what we are doing or contemplating, which will keep us right where we are (for better or worse); or, push through to achieve a new normal.

There are tools in the next two chapters to better determine whether we are bound for the "Stop!" path or the "Go For It!" path. For now, though, let's think about where this guidance comes from when we are faced with discomfort. Is it

Divine Guidance from some greater intelligence, our own intuition based on past experience, or our best guess?

It could be any of those things, based on our spiritual, religious, scientific, or personal views. 12-Step programs assist addicts of all types on the road to recovery. They share a common belief in the concept of a "higher power." The programs don't, however, determine for the addict what she or he identifies as their higher power. For the religious it means God, G*d, Jesus, Mohammed, Vishnu, Allah, or any number for other names of the Divine or a master teacher, prophet, sage, or guru. For the agnostic or atheist, who either believes God exists and does not care or is nonexistent, there is a completely different higher power. The guidance for these people may come from science, the beliefs of their family of origin, or the strength of a group itself, meaning the long-time members who have years of understanding and success in fighting the addiction.

A good example of what our use of intuition could look like is to compare human intuition to animal instincts. The beasts of the planet can't help doing what they do, or so we commonly assume. They're driven by impulses we assume can't be ignored. Suppose there's more to it? Consider the words of Dennis Merritt

Jones, from his book, *The Art of Uncertainty: How to Live in the Mystery of Life and Love It:*

> *At the level of animal, there is no real free will. Instinct will always lead an animal in a direction toward its survival. The same intelligence is working through human beings as intuition, broadcasting its "guidance beam" to all of us 24/7. The primary difference between the animal kingdom and ourselves is that animals don't have an ego to get in the way, and we do. The disadvantage of free will is that we also have the ability ignore the guidance that is being offered* all *the time. This is paramount information to embody as you navigate your way through the mystery of uncertainty. You are always at choice* (Jones, 2011).

What if our inner feelings, our intuition, is our best guess? What if we're making it all up? Here's a newsflash: We ARE making it all up! Deciding what we want our lives to be – where we go, what kind of work we seek, the relationships we form, and so much more – is all the result of the choices we make. The destiny in which we find ourselves is the culmination of making a variety of choices at various times. Even refusing to choose is a choice. If you or I refuse to make a choice then, in essence, that decision is a choice to take whatever we get or allowing someone else to decide for us.

If some or all of these concepts are foreign to you, this might be a good place to stop for a few minutes.

Taking time to consider what intuition means to you can determine your next step in healing some issue in your life. Get out a sheet of paper or your journal and a pen. I recommend you write down your thoughts, questions, or answers. The physical act of writing unleashes a different area of our brain, as opposed to typing on a computer keyboard or laptop. Give the following questions some thought:

Which of these three ideas about intuition (Divine, instinct, or personal direction)
resonate with you and why?

How has intuition, or the lack of it, demonstrated in your life?

Are there any childhood ideas about God wrapped up in a religion or belief system you no longer practice that could be at the core of discomfort you are experiencing in an area of your life?

Pain sensors are warnings

Our bodies have within them various types of sensors. Our sense of touch allows us to determine when an object is hot and when the same object is cold. This is true of all the objects we see, foods we taste, sounds we hear, and scents we smell.

No one needs to be told the difference in smelling our favorite flower and being acutely aware a skunk is nearby. We don't question those determinations – they are automatic based on past experience. Likewise, the pain sensors in our skin tell us when we can continue what we're doing or stop immediately.

Our bodies and the thoughts in our mind react the same way to non-physical situations. New ideas, suggestions by others, or meeting someone for the first time can cause us to become quickly aware something has changed within us to indicate caution. Those same things can give us the "Damn the torpedoes, full steam ahead!" response.

The question is, How do we know the difference when discomfort is involved? Does discomfort mean stop what we're doing or thinking about doing? Or does it indicate our ego is activating some kind of defense mechanism? Is our ego against a change of some kind because discomfort is necessary for us to move through and beyond our experience at the time?

The next two chapters offer ways to help you determine which of these two scenarios are being presented. Before continuing, consider completely these suggestions.

Now is another great opportunity to stop. Write down a few more thoughts that may be percolating in your mind. Ask yourself questions to which you want answers.

Record your emotional responses.

Give whatever you call intuition full permission to go for broke!

Chapter Three

When Discomfort Means "Stop!"

Our bodies are designed with nerve endings developed to provide pleasure and pain responses. The same action might cause different sensations depending upon the person or situation. Getting a foot rub, for example, is the ultimate pleasure for one person. Someone else might find it annoying because her feet are ticklish. Individually we might enjoy a physical sensation today that wasn't something we liked in the past. This shows the same feeling can change depending upon the situation, our mood, or the passage of time.

Physical pain isn't the only warning system our bodies possess. Our mental health is yet another way we're informed about an act or situation. There are probably people in your life who you look forward to seeing because being around them feels good. Conversely, you may feel depressed, fearful, or anxious if you anticipate having to interact someone else around whom you feel uncomfortable.

A Warning Sign of Real Danger

There are some noticeably clear examples of when discomfort is a warning sign of real danger. The pain we feel when attempting to lift a hot skillet off the stove without a potholder is a stark warning. We're being mindful about what we're doing.

If we hold onto a hot object of any kind for too long our skin will begin to redden and blister. We need to back off, get a potholder or gloves, and proceed. The same is true about the blaring sound of a siren which warns us of an approaching emergency vehicle; a caution sign that the bridge we are planning on taking has been washed out; or, the "DON'T ENTER" sign on the entrance to the cage of a wild animal.

All those warning signs make sense. You and I would rightly take notice of those and act accordingly to protect ourselves or others. What about the less obvious signs of discomfort? When do those mean to stop as opposed to pressing on? The following sections address various types of discomfort or pain in some common areas of life. They will also lay a foundation for the basis of the next chapter about how to know discomfort is a sign to go forward.

Health: Our Physical limitations

The elderly aren't the only ones growing old. Some of us are born with physical challenges. From infancy we're moving toward our eventual transition from this life into whatever we believe comes after what we're experiencing now. In other words, physical pain is no respecter of persons or age.

Even if we don't have an abundance of challenges today with our bodies, we may at some point in the future. The young, thinking they're invincible, are fearless. As we age, however, we discover to our chagrin this isn't the case. We often hear aches and pains poo-pooed by other people, even some health practitioners, because of our age. Bifocals are assumed to be needed when we reach our forties. Menopause, arthritis, loss of muscle tone, sexual dysfunction, and so many other ailments don't surprise us as we age because we're told to expect them.

Men and women alike frequently disregard the pain they suffer assuming it's one of the reasons above or countless other conditions about which they shouldn't be alarmed. This is especially true of women with regard to heart attacks. If you're like most people, the term heart attack immediately conjures up a picture of a middle-aged or elderly, possibly obese, male. The symptom is obvious: Excruciating chest pain.

This isn't necessarily true for females. The Worcester heart attack study, as reported in *The American Journal of Cardiology*, stated women didn't present with chest pain (Milner, Vaccarino, Arnold, Funk, & Goldberg, 2004). Because this common symptom predominately occurs in men, pain or discomfort suffered by women are attributed to other medical issues, such as indigestion or muscle strain.

Additionally, the internet has brought with it an assumption we can find out anything via our keyboards or mobile device. Self-diagnosis can be dangerous for anyone, though at least one study indicated men are twice or more likely than women to access "[w]eb searches for professionally-undiagnosed medical conditions (White & Horvitz, 2009). This information makes sense. Many studies have proven men are less willing to seek medical attention than their female counterparts (Schlichthorst, M., Sanci, L., Pirlis, J., et. Al, 2016; Mansfield, A.K., Addis, M.E., & Mahalik, J.R., 2003).

Fortunately, in my case, the post-surgery pain I was having wasn't life-threatening or damaging to my body in any way. Each of us need to be mindful of pain becoming a way of life. Some individuals may have a high tolerance for pain. Men, in particular, seem to think bearing pain, even when they don't have to, is some kind of badge of honor. It's not.

Disregarding pain as a warning sign can lead to ignoring classic symptoms of more serious situations. If we're toughing it out on our own and realize it's become part of our identity, then we're probably overdue for a consultation with a professional. No one should have to continually live with the discomfort of pain.

Wealth: How We View Prosperity and Money

Do you always have plenty of money to spend, share, and save? If you just laughed out loud don't worry – a lot of people would. Money issues and financial problems are one of the main causes of disagreements, arguments, and divorce among married couples.

Money is only one aspect of our prosperity consciousness. My friend, Helen King, says she has few needs and less wants. How can that be? It's because she knows her needs are provided abundantly by a universe designed to support her. She's aware most of the wants in the world are a result of extremely effective advertising and marketing.

Mass attacks on our egos through advertising media cause much discomfort for so many people. It seems many products we buy are nearly obsolete before we leave the store. There's always a bigger, better, or newer thingamajig or gadget we're told everyone *must* have! We're promised better looks, abundant sexual attraction, and longevity if we apply the cream, get the car, or take the pill. Diets of all kinds promise to be the *final* answer to our weight or health problems, even though we can historically link new diets to old ones.

We can eliminate the immediate discomfort of lacking the newest shiny object by purchasing whatever is being pawned this week. The problem is we often turn to a credit card – our plastic passports to fun! – to obtain said object. Eventually the statements on our cards come in. Instead of resting calmly in the satisfaction of what we thought would fix whatever we felt was wrong, we are faced with the stark realization we haven't got enough to pay off the credit card, or even make the minimum payment. The result? *More* discomfort!

This isn't to say credit shouldn't be used wisely and prudently. Neither does it mean we shouldn't have nice things for ourselves and loved ones. If we're feeling some *thing* will relieve the discomfort of lack we feel, it would behoove us to step back to figure out why we're experience the discomfort in the first place.

Remember, when discomfort stops us from moving forward it doesn't mean we won't eventually buy the object. It means we need to stop and to take stock of our intentions and motivations in purchasing whatever it is we're considering.

Love: Our Relationships

Have you ever been in a relationship you knew wasn't right for you? Perhaps the discomfort you felt was an ache in your belly upon meeting your mate for the first time. It might have been a quiet, somewhat fleeting feeling you should turn and run in the opposite direction, even though you did the opposite and fell headlong into the other person's embrace.

Every one of us has an energy signature. There are people who say they can see auras of energy, and those emanations change due to our moods or physical wellness. Electrical impulses are occurring throughout our bodies all the time. Humans are similar to two magnets which can be attracted to or repelled from each other depending on how the two magnets approach one another. We're naturally attracted to or repelled from other people for reasons we can't always understand – it's "just a feeling," we say.

Our instincts of right and wrong, good and bad, or yes and no are far stronger than may be commonly thought. For some reason – perhaps our upbringing, religious beliefs, or lack of confidence – we can be almost eager to dismiss our own inner guidance, intuition, or gut reaction. Conversely, we may feel compelled to act on the advice of others or outdated ideas from our past, feeling someone else knows better than we do, or it's more comfortable to follow the same paths we've walked most of our lives.

If we feel discomfort around someone there may be a particularly good reason. It doesn't mean we should avoid the person or refuse to get acquainted. However, we might want to allow it to give us at least a cause for pause before we pursue a friendship or other kind of intimate relationship. People who believe in past lives or reincarnation have said we're drawn to people in this life who are our soul mates. We may be learning life lessons together or working out issues in this life which occurred in a life we don't remember.

That might sound a little more woo-woo than you're willing to entertain, or it could make complete sense to you. Whatever the case, there's a definite reason for the feelings we have upon meeting people for the first time. It might be they embody characteristics of someone in our recent or distant past whom we loved, or hated, or someone who abused us in some way.

It doesn't mean the person in front of us is the other person. Even identical twins can have completely opposite personalities. To judge a person as bad or unworthy of our affections because they look like, act like, or have beliefs like

31

another person whom we dislike isn't fair – not to the person before us or to ourselves.

Again, discomfort isn't always an "end of discussion, stop what you're doing" situation. It's a warning system or can be a "have you considered …." opportunity to reflect on our perceptions as appropriate for the circumstances or built on incredulous beliefs.

Full Self-Expression: Our Way to Express Life

Our jobs or careers often define who we are. Even the two words – job and career – are frequently used synonymously, yet they can have quite different meanings. When we move into retirement, a whole different scenario occurs regarding our identity. For this reason, this section is divided into two sub-sections: **Job and Careers**, and **Retirement and Hobbies**

Jobs and Careers

There are differences between working at a job and having a career. A job is performing some act or producing a product in exchange for money and other compensation.

Hopefully, the work is at least tolerable if not enjoyable. Sadly, this isn't always the case. A career, on the other hand, is a life course, the way we express our unique gifts and further our interests. Not everyone working at a job is miserable; nor does it mean career-oriented individuals are delighted with every part of their work life. There are probably as many people who feel stuck in a dead-end career as there are people living paycheck to paycheck in jobs without meaning or fulfillment. The question is, Why?

We might have thought the career we're in was what we wanted to do. Then, after years of education (accompanied by outrageous student loans balances) and a considerable length of time in our field, we may find we still aren't happy. We regret spending so many years of training only to find out we don't like the field. This is a situation which can become unbearable. Some people stay where they are because their parents wanted them to become a doctor, or attorney, or something else, and they don't want to disappoint mom or dad.

Many years ago, when I was living in West Hollywood, California, fusion cuisine was becoming all the rage. Unlike today there were very few fusion restaurants back then. One opened up right across the street from where I worked. The place was doing excellent business and turned out to be lucrative for the owner. The owner's story, however, was even more intriguing than the new cuisine.

The owner was an extraordinarily successful and high-powered attorney in Beverly Hills. One day, with the salary, the car, the corner office, and a great house he realized he hated his career. What he'd always wanted to do was own a restaurant. That wasn't the dream his parents wanted for him, so he went to law school and built a law practice. One day he became sick and tired of being sick of his work. He sold the practice, invested nearly all of his money into this newly evolving cuisine and followed his passion.

This man had the means to do this. Money was no problem. For the majority of people, however, leaving a job or career isn't financially feasible. Feeling unsettled where we are is more than likely a result of acknowledging discomfort, not necessarily acting on it immediately as did our restauranteur.

In this area of our life, discomfort is guiding us to re-evaluate our situation. It moves us to pause, to take stock, and then move forward with a plan of action. It would probably be unwise to quit our jobs or leave our career without any idea of what really floats our boat. We want to *act*, not be in a state of *reaction*. Without a clear conception of what will fulfill our passion and needs we have little chance of success. This discomfort, however, will lead us to a point in time when discomfort means "it's time," which is discussed in the next chapter.

Retirement and Hobbies

You might have heard someone say they just can't wait to retire and do nothing. Few, if any, successful retirements are without doing *something* (Gewoib, 2015). After years of working, even if we have loved what we did, doing nothing is unsatisfying in the long run. The book you are reading was being completed during the 2020 COVID-19 pandemic. This worldwide crisis brought us some interesting, if not eye-opening, opportunities.

This is not to say the pandemic is a good thing by any means. Sheltering at home, and perhaps being furloughed, fired, or made otherwise redundant at our jobs or careers has created an unscheduled break from our daily routines. We have the option, of course, of being in discomfort about the situation 24/7, which is exactly what many have chosen to do. Blaming our discomfort on governments and leaders is just as counterproductive as blaming our doctor for a longer than expected time for recovery.

Many people are using the time to accomplish projects around the house they've been putting off due to a busy work schedule. Others have found online language programs, which seem to be booming (Andress, Givant-Star, & Balshem, 2020). Some are saying with some amount of pride that they are "test driving retirement."

The discomfort one can feel in retirement can lead to more serious problems, documented thoroughly in medical and psychological journals for years due to the increase of depression and the physiological effects of untreated severe mental health problems. The discomfort we might feel in retirement could be interpreted as a sign of failure in our life. We might have expected to be without debt, carefree, and traveling the world. Instead, we may be concerned about yet another hospital procedure or home repair.

That same discomfort and discontent might show up in the hobbies and activities we used to love (but no longer pursue), or about the ones we start and find ourselves less than enthusiastic. We always said we'd learn to play golf, only had no idea how expensive the sport it can be. We might have admired a certain form of art, though discover we have no aptitude for it or desire to learn to paint or sculpt.

These feelings of discomfort in retirement and hobbies are *not* a sign of failure. This type of discomfort is a wake-up call something just isn't right. It's a time to pause, take a break, and reassess what it is we want to do with our lives and free time.

Spiritual: Connecting with the Divine

So far, we've covered the topics of health, wealth, love, and career. These are the four major areas of life. In my counseling practice over the past 30 years I can't think of one person who didn't come to see me about one, or a subset, of those topics. Spirituality, however, isn't an issue addressed as much in the field of mental health, although strides toward its inclusion have been made over the past decade.

Religion, spirituality, and prayer were not taught in this field 50 years ago. Today they're no longer taboo subjects. In fact, understanding a client's spiritual practices or religious beliefs, or that of their family of origin, provides an additional insight to their approach to dealing with the other four areas of life. That's why a fifth area of life, spirituality, has been included.

People are seldom raised without some participation in or knowledge of religion. It's said about religious institutions, "The only thing bad about organized religion is that it's organized." Most religions are sure their practices are the only, or at least the best, ones to connect with God.

Religious wars and strife have plagued humankind for millennia. All efforts to subjugate or convert those of a faith different than our own have been disastrous, ending in heartache and death for hundreds of millions of people.

It all comes down to an "I'm right, you're wrong," attitude seen in religion, politics, business, and everyday life. One of the easiest ways to stop an argument is to agree with the other person. Doing so completely takes the wind out of their sails. This works well for disagreements between individuals, nations, and religious zealots. What about when we're having those discussions with ourselves? If one was raised with strict religious beliefs and left the faith, disobeying those rules and regulations adhered to by the faithful can be extremely uncomfortable.

How can discomfort with regard to faith in God, some higher power, or the lack thereof mean we should stop doing what we're doing? Shouldn't religious and sacred rituals bring us satisfaction and peace, not discomfort and anxiety?

Ideally, they would. Often, however, those rituals may no longer support who we are today. All religions claim they lead to God, heaven, nirvana, or some other reward. How can that be true when the numerous religions are so diverse and some diametrically opposed to one another?

Discomfort with our spiritual connection to God or something greater than ourselves isn't a reason to stop what we've been doing for most of our lifetimes. However, it's a good indication we should pause, reflecting on why our beliefs or actions are causing discomfort. If the root of discomfort is guilt about not pleasing our parents or a religious organization, then this cause for pause is probably indicative of a far greater issue.

Guilt and shame are experiences we feel throughout our lives. Both can be useful tools in healing, as long as those emotions aren't allowed to run rampant. If we've committed a crime or intentionally hurt someone guilt is obvious. The related emotion to guilt is shame, the feeling of remorse or regret at having harmed another or done something we know to be wrong.

Acknowledgement of our guilt and the experience of shame are healthy responses to situations for which we're responsible. What isn't healthy is when guilt and shame become toxic. Women who were raised to be subservient to men often apologize when they've no need to do so. This doesn't apply solely to women, of course. There are plenty of men who have an ingrained attitude about making everything right for everyone. And, should something go amiss, it's they who must immediately take responsibility by apologizing for something over which they had no control in the first place.

Now, lest you think we have casually left the area of the spiritual concept of allowing us to feel comfort with the Divine, let us apply these experiences of guilt and shame to religious belief. Even though we may have determined years ago the religion of our youth no longer connects us spiritually with something greater than ourselves, going against the rules of one's faith of origin may still cause a twinge of guilt or shame.

Though this can be subtle on the surface, it gives us a window into unresolved thoughts and beliefs we still hold sacrosanct. Here's how a situation such as this could look: A former practicing Catholic might insist on eating only fish on Fridays during Lent, even though he doesn't observe Lent; a person who was raised as one of Jehovah's Witnesses might feel awkward when she stands for the national anthem or pledges allegiance to the flag of her nation; or others might experience these feelings when they celebrate or observe a particular holiday which wasn't a part of their upbringing.

Feeling discomfort with regard to spirituality isn't a stop sign to cease our current actions in favor of the way we might have been raised. It is, however, an amazing opportunity to reexamine our beliefs, our faith, and our connection to a higher power. It's a loving reminder we've given ourselves to stop and acknowledge we might still have a bit of work to do on our consciousness and our beliefs. Our lives today may be drastically incongruent with the way we were raised, i.e., a lesbian and her wife are probably not going to be seen as a Mormon in good standing by their local ward. It's up to us to decide in which world we will live, the one we are told is right, or the one in which we feel we can express our own unique divine nature. As we become more comfortable doing one or the other, instead of continuing to straddle the fence between the two, the less discomfort we will feel with our spiritual connection and our actions.

This chapter has discussed discomfort in five different, yet interconnected, areas of our lives:

- Health: Our physical limitations
- Wealth: How we view prosperity and money
- Love: Our relationships
- Full self-expression: Our way to express life, made up of jobs and careers, or retirement and hobbies
- Spirit: Connecting with the Divine

Our discussion has been centered on allowing discomfort to mean you and I should stop what we're doing before making any major changes in our lives. The next chapter will review the five areas of life again, this time from the perspective of when the discomfort means to act. And, quite often, act definitely and with mindfulness. This is another good time to stop or pause, to allow thoughts to sink in. Grab that journal or paper again and begin to distill what we've cover so far.

Take a look at the five area just listed.

Which one jumps out at you?

Ponder any questions you have.

How do the concepts apply to your own life?

Has there been a time in your life where some issue has brought you to a complete halt?

Continue through the list until you've written something about each of the five areas.

Finally, take a few, quiet minutes to yourself. Close your eyes and ask what is next for you. Allow the answers to come gently. Force nothing. Even if nothing comes to mind, know that your life is unfolding in perfect and divine right order.

Chapter Four

When Discomfort Means "Go For It!"

O ur minds are so fantastic in the way they work for us. Have you ever had the experience of hearing just one phrase of music or noticing a scent, only to find your thoughts filled with memories? Other times an offhanded comment of a friend can spark a barrage of thoughts, recollections, or ideas.

This is what happened to me when Dr. Barsanti first admonished me to use discomfort as my guide. I was immediately conflicted. My mind raced back to 1983 soon after Nautilus gym equipment first came out. I was urged to push myself on a chest machine by a trainer. My inner voice said, "Uh, not a good idea, Terry." My male ego wanted to show the trainer I was made of firmer stuff and went for it.

I wasn't the wisest move I'd ever made. I tore a muscle in my left shoulder. It stopped me from working out for weeks.

I find working out, whether in a gym or at home, to be invigorating. There are physiological and biological reasons why you and I feel better when we are active. I was anxious to get back into being more physically active again after my hernia surgery. I wondered what my rule of thumb could be to stretch my limitations and not injure myself in the process. This led to my differentiating between the ego and a term which comes from a passage in the King James Version of the Bible (1 Kings 19:12). This phrase is used extensively by the Transcendentalist and New Thought movements of the U.S., which began using it in the 19th century: *the still small voice.*

When I was in my first years as a ministerial student one instructor stated God doesn't usually scream at us with the answers to our requests. There are subtle hints, signs around us if we're conscious of them, so in essence a still small voice. Other ways of understanding this is to consider it to be our intuition, a powerful tool in our lives if we're willing to learn to trust it. Just to clarify, however, in speaking about the still small voice it's not suggesting that we will or should literally hear a voice. Rather, it's a metaphor for the gentle way in which we can be guided to our highest good without the drama too often associated with change.

The focus of the previous chapter centered on how to trust our bodies and intuition when discomfort arises in our life. As we move into the area of relying on those same signals we first need to set the stage for why our first inclination would be to stop what we're doing, even though at the same time we feel pulled to do the exact opposite. To accomplish that we'll look at how *fear* plays a large part in our decision about whether or not *to push through* anything standing in the way of our next actions. To help us in that regard, the concepts of *mindfulness, common sense,* and *change* will be examined to complete a set of practices necessary to understand when moving forward is in our best interests.

Fear From Our Ego

The emotional and physical responses we experience from our ego are fear-based discomfort. I pushed through the chest machine at the gym because my ego thought the trainer would think I was a wimp if I didn't. At that time in my life how I appeared to others was more important to me than following my own intuition and being the person I was meant to be.

It has been said fear is the underlying feeling of all other emotional experiences we judge as negative or undesirable. This is especially true of anger. When we get mad at someone, we usually find underneath the initial rage is disappointment. Next, we'll find sorrow or sadness, and finally at the very bottom, fear. Fear that because we disappointed our partner he will leave. Fear that because we didn't get the job we wanted we will not find anything else. It's an interesting process to work through and a valuable one as well. The process, however, may be accompanied by a good deal of discomfort. If we stay in anger mode without knowing the underlying cause (which frequently has nothing at all to do with the situation), there can never be a complete healing of the situation. An unwillingness to do this work and to forgive other people and ourselves ruins our relationships. Eventually, over the years, it can be a catalyst to severe health issues, both mental and physical.

Pushing Through

It's by learning to trust our intuition that you and I can know when discomfort means to stop what we're doing as opposed to when it means to push through to reach a goal or affect change in our life. You might ask, How do we learn to trust our intuition?

Think back to when you were a child. Do you remember times when you knew something, accepted it was true, and later realized you didn't remember learning it? When you shared this information with an adult did you receive a response similar to, "Now how do you know that?"

Everyone has intuition. It isn't a quality some people possess, and others don't. Intuition isn't to be confused with clairvoyance. The latter is described as the supposed ability of a person to gain information about an object, person, place, or event through extrasensory perception. Conversely, intuition can be the capacity to remember something we may or may not realize we knew or observed in the first place. If you believe in a higher power, intention can also be considered a direct conduit of communication with the Divine. It's our ego who tricks us up about following this ability. Why?

Because the ego prides itself on figuring things out. Cultures often teach and pride themselves on the idea anything worth having is worth working for, and the harder we have to work the better. If we want something really, really, really, really desirable, then we must work really, really, really, really hard to get it. It's a given there will be sacrifice involved.

Intuition is the opposite. We know what to do, what path to follow, without any great deal of thought, sacrifice, or calculations about why we're certain we know a fact or answer to a situation. This throws the ego completely off kilter.

When adults may be surprised by a child knowing something they aren't expecting her to know, it might be the girl is accessing some tidbit of knowledge she heard from the TV, or in a conversation she overheard. Our brains take in far more information than we could ever imagine. What we remember is predicated on many issues, perhaps the most common is the importance it has to us. Importance to us is the clue. Four people can witness a car accident and the law enforcement officers taking the reports will most definitely not end up with identical accounts. This is why so-called eyewitnesses to crimes or accidents are often unreliable on the witness stand.

There are amazingly simple ways not requiring risk of physical harm or financial loss to increase our awareness of intuition. We can teach ourselves to know when and when not to allow it to influence our decisions. Perhaps you are driving to the store or to work and have a thought out of nowhere to turn down a different street than you would normally use. Most people will not follow through on that. Why? Because our egos thrive on consistency. Consistency is the illusion that there is no change – more about this in the next section.

I can only give you my personal experience of this. When I've given these examples in seminars or workshops I've conducted, I frequently see a number of smiles and heads nodding. For example, finding a parking place in front of the store when everyone said it couldn't possibly be there. Or, perhaps driving by a billboard which is of no interest to me as far as buying the product or service, yet something on it triggers an answer to a question I had. It might be that I've decided to go to a different restaurant or coffee shop than I usually do only to run into a friend or start chatting with a complete stranger. In conversation, the person has set me on a different trajectory in solving a problem.

Mindfulness

Did I lose you, or are you one of the ones smiling and nodding your head? If you are the former, I only suggest you consider these ideas. There's no need to attempt to force these thoughts. Just be willing to invite them in. It can be as simple as being at the traffic light and thinking, Should I go left, or right? As long as the light is green and the crosswalk is clear, make the turn you first thought of. No telling what you will find!

These ideas of being more aware of our thoughts is part of the practice of *mindfulness*. The practice has received much press in recent years, though the concepts of mindfulness are nothing new. Buddhism, yoga, and other philosophies have incorporated meditation into their belief systems or taught mindfulness in some form or another for thousands of years.

We live in a world demanding our constant attention. This isn't, however, necessarily for our health and well-being. Much of what we see, hear, and read is designed to get us to buy something we are being convinced we need. The way technology and mobile devices have grown exponentially in recent years has increased our practice of turning our attention to a screen on some device instead of other people or our surroundings.

Common Sense

If you are still skeptical, and even if you are not, another way to recognize intuition and the effects of practicing mindfulness is what most people call common sense. The brain seems to be capable of coming up with solutions to issues or problems drawing on previously experiences, many of which we may have forgotten on the level of our day-to-day awareness. Often it amounts to the common sense we've been taught over the years. We didn't necessarily acquire this ability by sitting down to consciously learn something. Rather, it was by observing the outcomes which occurred from our decisions, or what we saw unfold in the lives of others.

You may already have thought of an example of this in your own life. If not, let me share another painful one of my own. I've left a top drawer open while I went searching for something in a lower one far more often than I care to admit. On my way down I think, "I should close the drawer, so I don't hit my head on the way back up. Naaahh … I'll remember." I don't. So, I crack my head open, start bleeding, end up with a gash in my bald head, and get a headache to boot as a reminder to myself of my inability to learn by experience and follow my intuition. This is further exacerbated when people ask what I did, I tell them, and (shaking their heads scornfully at me) say, "You should know better," or "You should be more careful." Duh!

Accept these inner thoughts as intuition, a still small voice, your guardian angel looking out for you, mindfulness, common sense, or anything else you want. Science is only beginning to scratch the surface of what it means to fully comprehend how our brains operate. Our consciousness develops in marvelous ways over the years without us having to think about it doing so. If we're aware of what's being shown to us we'll be better equipped to decide how or if to incorporate the information in our lives.

Little Change Without Discomfort

I promised you in a previous section I would talk more about consistency in our lives being an illusion. The ironic truth is:

The only constant in life is change

On planet earth we are born, we live, and we die. The changes between the time we are born and the time we are placed in a casket are too numerous to count. The life we experienced this morning is gone, never to be replicated. Yes, we may go through the same motions, but the coffee might not be as hot, or the toast buttered to our expectations. Couples may often go back to the restaurant where they met to celebrate their anniversary. It isn't going to be the identical in all aspects. As long as they focus on the reason for being there instead of the fact the restaurant redecorated in some horrible fashion, or the menu is different, they will be fine. It's being together that's important. A different wall color or an item missing from the menu shouldn't ruin their evening.

When discomfort comes from change in our lives it might be partially caused by our unwillingness to celebrate loss. Now why would we celebrate loss? Think of being an undergrad for four years, then immediately continuing on to a three-year graduate program. If we count 12 years of elementary, middle, and high school, the graduate who walks across the stage just finished 19 years of school. That is definitely something to celebrate. How can there be loss?

It's a loss of identity. For the past 19 years she has been a student. In the time it takes to walk across the stage, shake hands, receive her degree, everything changes. No longer is she a student. After nearly two decades of one identity she is expected to change immediately. It is expected she'll find work, pursue a career, and perhaps begin a family if she has not already done so.

Does this make sense to you? If not, ask anyone who had been married for a long period of time and then divorces or loses a spouse in death. My mother is nearly 90 years old and for the past couple of years has lived alone for the first time in her life. At age 16, she went from my grandparents' home into a marriage with my father, divorcing almost 34 years later. She wasn't alone after the divorce, as my sister was still living at home. Two years later she remarried and my stepfather died after they had spent 35 years together. At 85 years of age she was faced with redefining who she was as a single, independent woman. That is change. And, in case you are wondering, it was definitely change for the better in spite of the circumstances. I've never seen her so alive and full of joy.

There will always be a little discomfort (or let's face it, sometimes a lot) when big change enters our lives. We can stay stuck in the present, pining for what was, or we can push forward and through the discomfort to a different and conceivably better situation. The great plus point about whatever decision we make is this: We can always choose again. Yes, this also means change ... again. And, yes, it might be accompanied with more discomfort. We can be a victim of our circumstances and stay stuck, or we can forge ahead empowered in knowing we have what it takes to create a life worth living.

Health: Our Physical limitations

Physical pain is probably one of the most debilitating experiences in human life. It doesn't matter if the pain is caused by an accident of some kind or it's the aches and pains we experience due to overexertion or aging. It sucks. It means we can't run around and play with our grandchildren the way we'd like to do. It stops us from going out with friends to dance or play sports. Pain becomes the deciding factor when we consider taking an extended vacation.

When most people consider the term "health" what comes to mind is the physical aspect of health, how our bodies are working, or how they aren't working. There's another aspect of health above and beyond physical limitations. Our mental health and emotional outlook are equally important to consider.

The level of our physical and mental health is far more intwined than we might think. A person who is normally happy, peppy, and the life of the party, can become depressed and despondent if faced with physical limitations and chronic pain.

Intense or prolonged pain can be terribly difficult to push through. The inability to move without discomfort can easily cause us to want to give up. Why start something we're sure we can't complete? An underlying concept throughout this book is how our attitude affects our daily activities, as well as our lives in general. Almost nothing has the effect of stopping us like physical or emotional pain.

Yet pushing through the pain is exactly what we may have to do. The question becomes, "Do I want to live fully, or do I want to give up?" Think about some accomplishment in your own life. Did it come easily to you? A person doesn't just wake up one morning and think, "Yep! Gonna earn my PhD today."

While this is outrageous example, I hope you get the point. Most of the accomplishments in our life require at least some effort on our part. Few things are handed to us on the proverbial silver platter.

Sure, gifts are nice, and there are plenty of people we can think of who seem to have everything given to them without any effort. Usually, however, the reality is often the opposite. Few people are "over-night successes." The fact that most performers struggle for years perfecting their craft is completely ignored when fame finally catches up with all the preparation and hard work. We don't have to struggle with every task. Even a little effort on our part produces a type of satisfaction we can't get from a chore being done for us. It seems to be encoded in our human DNA to want to work out our problems. Why? Because it empowers us.

This section isn't about giving medical advice. Nor will it suggest anyone cease taking medications or treatments designed to alleviate pain without first checking with the professionals who prescribed the drugs or suggested a particular regimen. We must speak with our health professionals. Having open, honest, and perhaps blunt conversations with our medical providers can be the first step to taking charge of our own healing processes. They can't help us if they don't know what's going on.

Obviously, I advocate this plan. The whole reason this book came into being was the attitude-changing conversation I had with Dr. Barsanti about the pain I was experiencing. Our conversation happened after I made an appointment *and showed up for it.* For some reason people often know they need to see their doctor, schedule an appointment with the office, but then no-show or find a reason not to go. I wasn't receiving weekly calls from Dr. Barsanti's nurse, Barry, to see if I was okay, nor would I have expected him to do so. If the discomfort of any procedure or situation continues or gets worse, patients must reach out.

Consciousness as a society is shifting. No longer will most people be satisfied with going to the doctor, having her tell us what to do, and then following instructions. Instead, we seek out an experienced, kind, and compassionate physician, nurse, or other healthcare professional who want to walk with us on a path to healing. We choose these particular people because we trust their expertise and counsel. They're willing to partner with us to facilitate our healing by working with our individual situations and giving us the tools to do so.

If you're experiencing physical or emotional pain, please reach out. There isn't anything to be ashamed of in seeking help. In the meantime, refuse to focus on pain stopping you from doing what you want to do. Turn your attention to whatever you *can* do. You might not be able to run a marathon. Could you walk (even with assistance) to your mailbox? You may not be able to bench press your own weight. Could you learn some stretching exercises to promote flexibility? Would a strength building program be possible for you using the very lightest of weights to start?

Physical pain and depression triggered by emotional issues work the same way. We might be very distraught about the death of a loved one, losing our job, or being dumped by the love of our life. Dwelling on the sadness of these situations year after year won't make us feel any better or change anything. Neither will spending hours crying over our departed years after their passing or spending time brooding about the boss we're sure hated us.

At some point it's time to let discomfort be our guide and push through the sadness and disappointment. Only we can determine when that time arrives. To quote a dear friend of mine:

You've suffered long enough.

Are you willing to try something else?

Wealth: How We View Prosperity and Money

What we focus on increases. That doesn't mean staring at our wallet hoping for more money will cause the bills to magically appear. It does mean, however, whining about not having any money, or constantly telling everyone how poor we are, will aid in perpetuating the very experience we claim to despise. "What we focus on increases" works both ways. Additionally, it's really a bore and quite draining to be around anyone like that, don't you think?

Wealth is far more than just money. It's about having an abundance of whatever we individually value. There are plenty of people who live simply yet lack for nothing. Conversely, there are others living in mansions whose lives are centered on getting more, and more, and more, with no real satisfaction in sight, surrounded by families who barely know them.

Even though wealth goes beyond having money, it's important to acknowledge cold hard cash plays a major role in the lives of most of us. Money in and of itself is a basic means of exchange. We don't think of currency, debit cards, credit cards, or any of the other ways we pay for purchases as bartering. It is. Someone has something we want and we barter with cash in some form. It could be they have a chicken we want and we have a couple of bales of hay that they want. In modern society we very seldom find our lives working this way.

There's a kind of discomfort we can feel about money and it means "Go for it." This has to do more with the emotional attachments we have about financial or wealth-building actions, such as investing or saving. If something sounds too good to be true it probably is. The discomfort we feel around such offers is a sure sign to stop considering the purchase or investment.

What feels right to us can also bring up discomfort. Why is that? We may still have outdated beliefs around money, finances, and prosperity, ones common to our upbringing or culture. For example, some years ago I read an article indicating we can hit a financial barrier when we reach the point in our lives where we meet or exceed the wealth or station in the lives of our parents. This may or may not be your experience. If it's true for you there can be a bit of a twinge which is definitely discomfort. We're more comfortable, they're proud of us, and we still might feel "off." Why?

If we looked to our parents as examples, a gold standard of success if you will, equaling or surpassing their financial station in life might create an uncomfortable feeling of unworthiness. If mom and dad couldn't get to my level of wealth, why do I feel I deserve it? Will my success make them feel like they failed to provide us with what we deserved? This certainly isn't true of all of us, but this consideration can provide insight into our beliefs around wealth.

We don't have the lives or financial prosperity we deserve. We have the lives or financial prosperity we *think* we deserve. Saying we deserve a material possession, status, or a financially comfortable life doesn't mean we *believe* we deserve it. The first time I considered this idea it resulted in my ego throwing himself to the floor kicking and screaming. How dare anyone suggest such a thing! Yet there is a golden thread of truth in this theory throughout all areas of life.

This idea may not resonate with you. Like the rest of this book, I'm offering suggestions to having a life worth living. Not the life we *think* we should have, the life we *want*. Give it some thought. Or not. Let discomfort be your guide!

Love: Our Relationships

Leaving an uncomfortable or harmful relationship can be tremendously difficult. This is a part of life upon which you and I would do well to trend lightly in some instances, and face head on in others. Let's look at the latter part of this situation first, as it's the more volatile and potentially dangerous.

If you are in a physically, sexually, emotionally, or psychologically abusive relationship you must act as quickly as possible to change the situation. No one deserves to live a life of misery due to the abuse of others. This doesn't necessarily mean to walk out of the house today, tomorrow, or next week. It's a wake-up call to get help now!

Walking away from a relationship without healing what needs to be handled can be a double-edged sword. As difficult as it may be to believe with regard to relationships, something in our consciousness draws people to us and us to them. Perhaps we don't feel we deserve better. Most of the time what's continually drawing abusive or angry or unsatisfying people into relationship with us is completely unconscious on our part. Uncovering such a pattern may require professional help to heal the issue and move on. This isn't to say we are at fault or to blame. There is no God above forcing lessons on us, at least not in my belief system. The higher power in which I trust is a non-judgmental, ever-present force, always there to support us, *if* we allow it to do so.

Refusing to release the past and current discomfort of trying to put the square peg in the round hole will only re-create another relationship of the same kind. No one wants that, which is in and of itself is an extremely desirable reason to stop ignoring a pattern and learn how to change it.

The "treading lightly" part of the discomfort often means whatever discomfort is coming up might very well be due to the fact we are not expressing something in a relationship we need to express. We might be afraid our partner will be angry, or we'll hurt their feelings. Learning to approach our partners with loving compassion while owning our own feelings is crucial in coming to agreement with them.

One major tool in doing this is speaking in the first person. We could say, "You make me feel like I'm worthless." Instead, if we phrase the communication to be about our own emotions it would more like, "I feel worthless when you ignore the work I've done around the house." Do you see the difference?

It means we take responsibility for our own emotions instead of blaming our partner. It was Eleanor Roosevelt who said:

No one can make you feel inferior without your consent.

This is true of many other emotional situations above and beyond inferiority. When we consistently and automatically live day after day and week after week with the same nagging issues in a relationship we are giving our partner the power to determine how we are going to feel.

On the flip side of the coin of relationships, what if a person has come into our life and wants to move forward, and we aren't sure about it? Are we excited or are we feeling a certain amount of discomfort? First, let's establish that spending the night or whole weekend together with someone we're dating is a whole lot different than agreeing to get married. Keep the situation in perspective.

Second, ask the discomfort (yes, you can talk to your feelings and talk to your body!) what the problem is, or why the discomfort is there. You *will* get a response in your thoughts. With this newly found information, ask yourself:

Is this true?

Then, How do I know this is true?

Next, If it has been true in the past is it really true now?

And finally, If it is true now, is this the way I want to continuing living?

Just because we had a bad experience in a similar circumstance sometime in the past doesn't mean the same outcome will be true for the current situation.

We can take comfort in knowing this doesn't have to be a "Yes" or "No" situation. It can be, "Maybe," which could be expressed as, "Wow, what an opportunity! Would you be willing to let me think about it and get back to you?" Put a time limit on it for yourself and the other person. The response you receive will also be a great determinator for you in coming to a satisfying decision.

Full Self-Expression: Our Way to Express Life

In the previous chapter this section was divided into our self-expression during the time in our lives when we have been working full-time, and a time allowing us more freedom to enjoy our inner desires to express in ways that may or may not result in financial benefit. While we might think of these two sections as working years and retirement years, it's not necessarily the case. Some people work at a job giving them the means to support hobbies and pursuits of interest to them. Others may have ceased a regular job and created a life in which they feel free to live without the expectation of a boss or business responsibility by developing a business of their own. How these next two sub-sections apply to you will depend on where you are personally in your life and desires.

Job and Careers

Both jobs and careers can feel unfulfilling or be a terrible burden in some way. The first thought some may have would be to leave the situation. That's not always the best idea for a number of reasons, not the least of being having the financial means to support oneself.

Leaving our career or job can be remarkably similar to leaving a romantic relationship. If we don't heal the stuff making us crazy around our work situation then "doing a geographic" (moving to a new city, area, or job to avoid the situation), as is said in 12-step programs, will not change the situation. Our unconscious seems to have an annoying ability to re-create the same types of disorganized boss or unhappy coworkers in the new position.

There can be an uncomfortable feeling about any change, A career or job change might require us to step up our game. We might be switching from labor to management. It could be taking our skills and training into a completely different line of work. Even accepting a salary far beyond what we've ever earned before can be daunting to some. Or it could just as easily be a career making us more excited than anything we've ever been offered, even though the annual income is lower than our present compensation.

When you and I are faced with discomfort in regard to our careers or jobs, we can ask ourselves some simple questions.

- Does the thought of taking this new job, starting this new career, or accepting this promotion absolutely excite me in ways I haven't felt before?
- When I first heard about this opportunity, did I immediately feel like a light went on?
- Did I have a "WOW!" moment or start to smile?

Too often our initial excitement is squelched by thoughts like:

- I'm not good enough for this.
- I don't have enough training.
- What if the people I'm supervising don't like me?
- I'm too old to start something new.
- People will laugh at me.
- What will other people think?

We could discuss why none of those thoughts or questions are a good enough reason for some not to go for it. Instead look at it this way. Would you be offered a promotion, a new job, or anything else by someone if they thought you would fail? Of course not. We are offered new opportunities because someone feels we can do the job, even if we have some doubts. It's good to understand, however, that just because we can, or someone believes we can, it doesn't necessarily mean we have to do it. The choice is ours.

As for what others think? Who cares! Plenty of people in their 50s, 60s, 70s, and even older have begun new careers or opened up to new interests only to find a niche offering happiness and fulfillment never before experienced.

Retirement and Hobbies

Retirement should be uniquely designed for each of us, not some cookie-cutter lifestyle imposed by societal or family expectations. Go back a page or two and re-think those questions posed about accepting a new job or career. They are just as applicable to our retirement or a hobby we might like to start.

Similarly, so are all the points listed above which could stopping us from moving forward. By the time we're old enough to retire we ought to have a clearer idea about how we want our remaining years to be spent. Hopefully, if we've chosen to spend our lives only pleasing others perhaps this is the time to begin living to see our own needs are met. Retiring doesn't mean getting ready to die. On the other hand, no one seems to be leading the way to living forever in the body we have. If you want to learn to crochet, start painting, or take a two-week jaunt up the Amazon and say, "No, don't think now is a good time," exactly when *will* it be a good time? There may not be that many shopping days left till Christmas, if you get my drift.

What does it mean when if we say, "I'm going to retire for the night?" It means we're going to bed, or at least somewhere near our bedroom, perhaps doing some reading before dozing off. It's not an indication we're going to start painting the bathroom or remodel the kitchen. It means we're going for a bit of rest. However, for some the idea of retirement can imply one is done living, as if she or he is retiring from life itself.

To combat this outdated idea of retirement we've come up with few new terms for this stage of life which are becoming popular. Neither of them indicates anything about winding down life. They are *re-wirement* and *re-energizement*. I've been using re-wirement for some time now, although I can't say it applies only to those of us who are 60-plus. This section presents re-wirement at any age when it comes to our jobs, careers, or the traditional retirement in society. Perhaps if we saw re-wirement throughout our life, retirement as we know it would be completely different. Instead of it being the end of our life it would be another transition, similar to all the other positive transitions we made throughout our life.

The other term, re-energizement, just makes me laugh. Not in a bad way, mind you. It might have been because the first person I heard it from is one of the most energetic women I know. When I think of my friend, Helen King, the first image I think of is the Energizer Bunny™. I can hardly keep up with her now and she's over two decades older than me.

Yet, like re-wirement, re-energizement is another practice we can start today regardless of our chronological age. You and I deserve a life we love. No one deserves to be miserable, wondering where the next meal is coming from, or worrying about where to live. No matter how successful we are in life there can be times when we feel stuck, in one form of discomfort or another, or can't quite put our finger on what's bothering us.

What a great time to do some self-imposed re-energizement! It could be a vacation, even a short one; a "play day" alone or with others; binge-watching a series; or many other things you may be thinking of which brings a smile to your face, activities you love to do, or something you've given up for some reason. Whatever method you decide to use, allow your discomfort in this area of life to catapult you into a more satisfying and enriching time.

Spiritual: Connecting With the Divine

Most people are raised with some knowledge of religion or religious beliefs. Some of us were taught religious principles at home, attended church or some other spiritual community, or might even have considered a type of ministry as a career. Attaining a personal connection with whatever we view as our higher power doesn't seem to happen for many people, even for the most faithful adherent to a religious organization or spiritual philosophy.

In the United States, an increasing number of people in recent years are identifying as "spiritual, not religious (Shaw, 2018)." Most of my clients who identify in this group have some kind of belief in a universal power or presence (maybe it's God, maybe it isn't), and that's about as far as it goes. There can also be an underlying feeling of "what if He *does* exist" from the patriarchal religious background from which many come.

The spiritual, not religious group definitely believe in God or some higher power. They just think S/He doesn't care. Some of them might be considered closet agnostics. Almost everyone in the spiritual, not religious category share a particular experience at the core of these feelings. Somewhere along the line, perhaps as children, maybe as a disenfranchised adult group, nearly all of these women and men feel organized religion failed them. It often turns out the religion didn't fail them. The same people may still have a desire to practice their faith. It was actions of a spiritual leader or members of the community who turned them away. As my Israeli friend, Amnon Shavit, said to me, "There is too much religion and not enough faith."

God, Jesus, Allah, or whatever we call the presence is often seen as an authority figure, not a best friend. Few people would consider God a lover. One of my teachers in ministerial school used to call God, "Big Sweetie." She had a complete love affair with her idea of God. She saw God as a presence totally supporting her, providing for her needs just like the Bible says God does, and never leaving her side.

Big Sweeter worked for her even though the designation might seem strange or completely out of context with your beliefs. She had an unshakable faith in her concept of God. That's exactly why she was able to trust her inner guidance.

It was in the rooms of Alcoholics Anonymous where the terms "higher power" or "God as we understood Him" became part of our culture. Not surprisingly, "the number of people who identify as 'spiritual not religious' has grown" in substance abuse groups just as they have in the general population, perhaps for the same reasons mentioned previously (McClure & Wilkinson, 2020). Terms like "higher power," "universal consciousness," "divine love," and many others don't have the religious history attached to them the way the word "God" has. These alternative terms are an effective way to embrace a type of comfort a person requires, without having to deal with the emotional baggage religion can create for us.

Even if you are an atheist or agnostic, aren't there times when you feel "sumpin' jus' ain't right?" It can be an uncomfortable feeling, the discomfort, which this whole book is about. Call it intuition, call it a gut feeling, or attribute it to scientific knowledge you acquired, or call it God, it's there in each of us.

The discomfort we might feel when we "just know something" even though we have no logical reason for thinking so can be an enormously powerful tool in making decisions. This isn't about how you and I feel about God, or even if there's a God. Rather it's how we feel about our inner guidance. Of course, if you have a strong belief in the God of your understanding, this still applies. Another example of this if you don't mind?

My mother is devout in her religion and raised me to believe as she does. I no longer share all those beliefs, though we still discuss matters of a spiritual nature. We've sometimes seen the exact same thing from two divergent positions. One day we were chatting, and she mentioned how strong the Devil is nowadays, how Christians must fight against all the temptations of the flesh more than ever before. "Excuse me," I said, "Did Jehovah suddenly lose His power? You taught me He was the Almighty, right?"

There was more than a little kerfuffle from her, and she responded, "Well of COURSE He is!" "Then why," I said as gently as possible, knowing it would get an adamant response, "don't you trust Him to protect you?" Her response is exactly what you're probably thinking. When the dust settled, she admitted that by challenging her faith I had reminded her of the power for which she has lived almost her entire life. It was, after all, she who taught me my personal beliefs should be able to withstand the test of fire, or in other words, being challenged.

It's taken over 30 years for us to get to a position where we can respectfully discuss spiritual topics that used to upset us both. I offer this story to you, particularly if you are a faith-based person, to encourage you to allow your faith in God to guide you in those times in which you feel discomfort. Trust in the God in which you say you believe. And, if you are not someone who believes in a higher power other than science or your own common sense, stop second guessing what you already know to be the truth for you.

Chapter Five

Implicit Bias

The term "implicit bias" has come into our conversations more frequently with the advent of #BlackLivesMatter and other movements focusing on discrimination, inequity, and inequality. It's not the purpose of this book to delve into those issues. The concept of implicit bias, however, is important for us to understand with regard to the pain and discomfort we might feel in any of the areas already examined.

What is implicit bias? In 2018, a team of three researchers publish an article in *Scientific American* about the term. They state it this way, saying "[it] sets people up to overgeneralize, sometimes leading to discrimination even when people feel they are being fair (Payne, Niemi, & Doris, 2018)." How does this apply to feeling discomfort in our own lives, or in our own thoughts?

In a completely different application, it goes back to that "sumpin' jus' ain't right" gut feeling we all have at one time or another. We don't know why we feel a certain way, but we have some strong feelings. Sometimes true emotional discomfort will arise about a decision, situation, person, or group of people. The way implicit bias works is extremely subtle. Our brains pick up all sorts of information throughout our lives. Most of the data isn't something we think about, though our brains store the information to be used later.

As we move through life information gets added to our inner database. Some knowledge goes into the long-term memory area of our brains because, for whatever reason, we stop using that information. Perhaps we begin to understand various situations or concepts differently than we have in the past. Eventually, we may forget all about them. The problem is, just like all the old, seldom-accessed files on the hard drive of our computer that we've never deleted, the old ideas are still there in our memory, not accessed anymore, but they still exist. Just as we could wrongly use an old, outdated file to create a current project, obsolete concepts or beliefs from our past can affect us if we allow them to do so.

This means our egos might jump back to those previous ideas we held so dear when we are presented with a new decision or opportunity. Even though it looks like green lights all the way, we might feel some discomfort based on those outdated experiences or data. It's important to be aware of these responses because we're all affected by implicit bias to one degree or another.

In the same article already cited, the authors go onto say, "One reason people on both the right and the left are skeptical of implicit bias might be pretty simple: It's not nice to think we aren't very nice." The way we were raised, "Little girls shouldn't do that," "Big boys don't cry," or "That's not very Christian," are all subtle ways we get programmed by our parents and society. Even though they were well-meaning in the way they instructed us, those ideologies don't work for us today.

It's important to understand implicit bias exists. It's not a judgment of whether you and I are good or bad, moral, or immoral, or anything else. Implicit bias is merely part of the equation. Should it cause us discomfort or pain, we can stop and analyze whether the warning is a valid one. In another context, we can ask ourselves what the *real* reason we are "swiping right" or "swiping left!"

Chapter Six

Looking Forward

This book is scheduled for publication late in 2020, a year that will forever be remembered as one of the most tumultuous periods in modern history. On the one hand we have seen more technological advances in the past fifty years than have been produced in thousands of years. The use of these advances in the scientific communities and in the palms of our hands exceed the current capabilities of our own brains. In other words, events and norms are changing quicker than ever before.

The challenges for true equality without regard for race, ethnic background, gender and gender identity, chronological age, and so many outward differences among the billions of inhabitants upon planet Earth give rise to a myriad of types of discomfort every day. How can we cope with the ever-changing world around us?

You and I must first realize we aren't here to solve the problems of the world tomorrow, nor is it necessarily our job to do so. True, a small number of us will be remembered in the annals of time as groundbreakers, liberators, and leaders of change. Most of us, however, must live with the realization that the memory of our lives may fade much more quickly than any of us might want to admit. Should this fact alone make us feel even more discomfort? That we'll never make a difference? That we have no purpose?

No, No, and No.

While you and I may never appear in a history lesson a thousand years or even a century from now, we can make noticeable differences every day to those around us and to the benefit of our world. The simple kindnesses we can show to one another and to complete strangers – and, yes, to those who appear to make it their purpose on earth to be hate-filled and rude – produce differences in the lives of people, the effects of which we'll never fully comprehend.

Giving a semi-trucker clearance to move over in front of us on the freeway, opening the door for someone even if they could easily do it themselves, returning a shopping cart for a fellow shopper, and a simple smile can totally change the energy of another person. In the process of "just being nice" we will find our own level of discomfort, irritation, and anxiousness lessen, while at the same time making someone else's life a whole lot easier.

Years ago, I was serving as the lead flight attendant in the first-class section of a flight going across country. I was the first flight attendant to greet the passengers and all was going along smoothly.

Until *she* got on the plane.

As soon as the smile appeared on my face and the words, "Good morning! Welcome aboard," were uttered all hell broke loose. "What are *you* so goddamn happy about?" Forget drop mic. I dropped jaw, recovered, and continued on. The woman was seated on the aisle in the first row of the cabin. When asking if I could offer the passengers a beverage, her response was not something I'll put in print.

I was taken aback, to say the least. I wasn't a newbie, someone just out of training or green at dealing with conflict. I thought to myself, *I am not going to deal with this for the next four hours. Period.*

I finished serving pre-departure drinks to everyone and walked back into the cabin. As the captain was finished her paperwork, I walked over to the woman, knelt down at her seat, and quietly explained that I attempted to do my job to the best of my ability. I said I took a great deal of pride in providing excellent customer service. As her mouth slightly opened to begin yet another barrage of insults and intimidation, I immediately said I didn't know what I had done for her to speak to me the way she had been since boarding, but if she would tell me I'd be happy to approach the situation better or make amends. I explained we had several hours to spend together and it was my hope we could make it as pleasant as possible for both of us.

The floodgates opened. I mean she bawled her head off. Within a few seconds I was holding her as she sobbed on my shoulders. I honestly can't remember, nor could I decipher, all the wrongs done to her or what she'd experienced over the past week. The day she had to travel by air she was required to navigate her way through security and the terminals at Atlanta's Hartfield International Airport while being pushed in a wheelchair. Suffice it to say that if something could have gone wrong it did.

Later during the flight she told me more. About the death of her husband, about the car breaking down on the way to the funeral, and the extreme sadness and anger she was feeling. She dealt with those feelings by being nasty and downright hateful to everyone around her, particularly to the people who appeared happy. She told me she considered herself a good Christian woman and was ashamed of her actions. She asked why I didn't snap back at her like everyone else did.

"Well, honey," I told her, "I reckon my mama jus' raised me right!" I thought she was going to wet herself. She smiled for the first time in days, started laughing so hard tears ran down her face, and by the end of the flight she was chatting and laughing with the other passengers around her.

Before she left the aircraft to get into the wheelchair waiting for her, she grabbed hold of me with the strength of one of those wrestlers on TV. She was quite an ample, older Black lady and I was a middle-aged rather tall, slender White guy. We must have been quite a sight to the agent meeting our flight in Las Vegas, as well as the captain saying goodbye at the cockpit door, neither of whom had any idea of what had transpired in the several hours.

I'm not trying to blow my own horn with this story. I offer it to you as an example of how a simple act of kindness can change *everything*. Have your ever heard the saying, "Practice random act of kindness and senseless acts of beauty?" The thought has been written out in various forms. The original is attributed to Anne Herbert who wrote an article entitled, "Random Kindness and Senseless Acts of Beauty." Her article "appeared in the July 1985 issue of the influential countercultural journal 'Whole Earth Review.'" Before that, however, the phrase, "random acts of kindness," appeared in 1951 London, when "'The Observer' published a radio drama appraisal that contained the distinctive phrase (Quote Investigator, 2017)."

With all due respect to Ms. Herbert or whomever originated this quote, I would suggest a change in her phrase due to the subject of our discussion here. What would happen, instead of practice *random* acts of kindness and *senseless* acts of beauty, we each individually began actively participating in practicing *intentionally loving* acts of kindness and *love-creating* acts of beauty?

Some might immediately say, "Well, not everyone would do it, so why should I bother to make the effort?" That reminds me of the answer my mother gave to a woman when she and I were engaging in door-to-door ministry. The woman at the door was ticked off because Jehovah's Witnesses don't serve in the military. "What would happen if *everyone* did that? Then where would the world be?" My mother's answer was not verbal. She just smiled, lovingly, quietly, and sincerely. The woman got it immediately and softened her attitude. If you don't *get* it, re-read the question and the non-verbal answer. You'll get it.

We can't control the actions of others. We can't force people to be upright, law-abiding citizens who care what happens to their neighbors. You understand when, in the beginning of this book, I said I would find it surprising to believe anyone reading this book doesn't suffer or hasn't suffered from some kind of discomfort. Don't we deserve for ourselves and family, to eliminate or at the very least alleviate as much discomfort in our lives and in the lives of the others around as we can?

I believe we do. You and I run into nasty, ugly, "I'm right and you're wrong," people all the time. What I can say from my personal experience is the less I mirror those kinds of attitudes, and the more I reflect the type of person I want to be, the fewer of those people seem to be around me. The concept of "what we focus on increases" was briefly mentioned early on in this book. Spiritual teachers, metaphysicians, and those who meditate know this. Science bears it out as well. Visualization, focusing on the act and the outcome of sports, came to light during the 1984 Olympics, when it was reported to have been used extensively by the Russian researchers. There are professional papers and studies available about how this applies to athletes, actors, and other performers. What those people have found in actual practice is visualizing their routines or acts, or regularly focusing on the completion of their efforts by receiving an award or prize, is just as crucial to their success as the physical act of practicing their sport or trade (Ekeocha, 2015; Newmark, 2012; Kumar, 2010).

These same principles work in our own lives as well. The practices of mindfulness, meditation, visualization, and personal empowerment were probably not part of your basic education in school. These modalities, among others mentioned in this book, all fly in the face of a modern worldview which says we must work physically hard to get ahead in life. Yet these ancient practices are being used more and more in schools, rehab facilities, and prisons (to name just a few areas) throughout the United States and other countries.

Dr. Taryn Reichard shared this thought after reading this book during the review stage: "There are pain psychologists to whom I will send my patients to help them learn these concepts. It really does make a difference."

Mindfulness isn't something that can only be accomplished sitting cross-legged, living in an ashram, or practicing vegan eating. We can be more mindful by giving life around us our full and undivided attention. How? Perhaps start by banning all cell phones at meals and having a meaningful dialog with each other. Remember that old saying about taking time to smell the roses? Do it. Stop, bend down, and breathe in the tantalizing aroma of a beautiful flower. Live each day in what I like to call *childlike wonderment*. Ever notice how kids can be laser focused on the simplest things? We adults can still do the same thing. It's fun, it lowers our blood pressure, and reduces stress.

Perhaps you've snickered at these seemingly childish or basic ideas. If that's you I must advise, "Don't knock it till you've tried it!" Most of us are living at hyper speed, barely noticing the many beautiful acts of kindness taking place around us all the time, focusing rather on the evening news and a steady stream of social media reporting the very worst of the worst ... repeatedly ... like over, and over, and over ... and over again. Is that the way you want to live your life? Constantly angry, fearful, or confused about world conditions and your future?

If after at least trying these easy ways to bring mindfulness into your own life you may want to up the ante. Yoga studios, massage therapy spas, and so many other businesses have trained and certified practitioners that can help you design a program suited to your lifestyle and schedule. These practices are not just for adults. In fact, the sooner we start to teach our children how to live in harmony with our planet and each other the better off we'll be.

One mindfulness meditation teacher in Dallas, Texas, Veronica Valles (ww.veronicavalles.com), has been teaching elementary-aged school children for a number of years with amazing results. The COVID-19 pandemic caused her to begin teaching mindfulness online, as well as providing one-on-one support for teachers and administrators in the public-school system. She recently said, "[The pandemic has] actually opened

the door to reach a variety of school districts from my home."
Veronica's work is her ministry to others and is one of countless
examples of how we can obtain the support we need regardless
of our situations.

Whatever course you choose to follow in your own
experience with discomfort in some area of your life tools are
available for your use. Reach out to professionals who are
qualified to assist you in getting back on a path to health,
happiness, and joy in your life. Above all, know you have within
you the power to change and release the discomfort in your life
that is keeping you from having a life worth living.

Discomfort is the call

to set yourself

free.

Byron Katie

Author's Acknowledgments

T he following medical professionals all reviewed the original draft of this book for medical accuracy and content, as well as their personal opinion:

My first acknowledgment and expression of appreciation must go, of course, to Ronald G. Barsanti, MD, my general surgeon (Pinnacle Health), for the excellent care he provided me, and for being the kind of caregiver everyone should have. Taryn M. Reichard, D.O. (Intervention Pain Management, Orthopedic Institute of Pennsylvania, and Arlington Orthopedics) for her expertise and guidance in assisting in my healing, and for the new friendship and honesty she so easily offers. Dayna Weinert, MD, (Assistant Professor of Integrated Medical Science, Florida Atlantic University, Charles E. Schmidt College of Medicine) a well-respected radiologist and professor, who just happens to also be the girl I loved in eighth grade – I'm so glad we've reconnected. Barry L Boyer, RN, Doctor Barsanti's office manager and nurse, whose tireless patience in answering my emails and making sure my family leave paperwork was processed, is appreciated more than he can possibly know. Dale Mausteller, RN, for additional medical information I didn't know I needed; and, whose keen eye and attention to detail saw more than one pothole that would have been rather embarrassing if it had gotten into print. Your support was amazing, but nothing compared to the friendship we have.

The original draft was also reviewed by a fellow minister and colleague, the Rev. Mary Ellen (m.e.) Cassey; fellow flight attendant (retired) and one of my closest friends, Debbie Roland; and, fellow author, Jo Anne Wilson. Ladies, *each* of you took the time to read and comment on this project. I have so much respect and admiration for you three. You each told me the truth, even if it wasn't what I wanted to necessarily hear. That's not simply good editing, it's the sign of a true friend! You are loved!

VIP Offer

I'm truly honored you read this book – thank you! If you enjoyed the book and would like to learn more about my work, there are a couple ways to do that.

Additional information is included in the next few pages. Some of those are links to my "Making Sense of Life" blog and how to find more books on a variety of subjects. Something not mentioned there, which is what I'll share with you here, are the benefits of becoming a subscriber to my email list.

As a subscriber, you'll receive a free eBook and a weekly email from me. The email includes an uplifting message and an affirmation for the week. You'll also be the first to know about other writings, new books that are coming out, online classes or talks I produce, where I might be speaking or holding a seminar in the future, and other "stuff" I only share with my subscribers. Finally, and this is a really cool part if I have to say so myself, each subscriber receives a free copy of future books just prior to their publication for the general market.

There's no obligation to sign up and you can unsubscribe easily if you choose to do so at some point in the future. To join this group of growing subscribers, go to my website at **terrydrewkaranen.com** and sign up! Thanks again!

Terry Drew Karanen

About the Author

Terry Drew Karanen is an award-winning author, freelance blogger, ordained minister, and at the time of this writing, still working as a professional flight attendant. He retired from 25 years of active ministry in 2019 after ending his fourth ministerial position. Terry holds a Doctor of Divinity degree in holistic theology from the American Institute and a Master of Social Work degree from Temple University. He uses his skills as a licensed social worker and spiritual leader through counseling, consulting, mediation, and conflict resolution. He has received advanced training as an employee assistance professional (EAP), advanced alternative directives (ADR) mediator, and as a critical incident stress management (CISM) counselor. His published articles and over 300 blog postings are available free of charge on his blog site, "Making Sense of Life" (blog.terrydrewkaranen.com) For a full catalog of all his available published writings, search "Terry

Drew Karanen" on Amazon.com, or visit his website at: **terrydrewkaranen.com**

Terry currently lives in south central Pennsylvania and travels the world for fun and for his professions. To book him as a speaker, seminar facilitator, consultant, or to schedule a virtual counseling session contact him through his website. Appointments are also available online through Square Scheduler, at: http://bit.ly/2JreEy2

Also by Terry Drew Karanen

Empowerment

From the Trailer Park to the Pulpit:
Reflections on the wise and wacky sayings of Grandma Esther

How to Find Your Vision and Get a Life! Using a vision and
mission to create a life worth living

Freedom to Live! Enjoying ease in four areas of life

It's Safe for Me to Be ...

Meditations for Life! Volume I (Originally published as
Treatments for Life!)

Meditations for Life! Volume II— The Wisdom of Women

Church Organization & Management

Beginning Your Own Work

Humor

The Beverage Service – A short story

The Res Book

"Making Sense of Life" Blog

blog.terrydrewkaranen.com

Most books are available on Amazon
(paperback and Kindle versions) at:
https://amzn.to/2Q8HdWa

References

Abraham-Hicks (Year unknown). Trust Your Instincts [Recorded by Abraham-Hicks]. Retrieved from https://www.abraham-hicks.com/

Andress, M., Givant-Star, M., & Balshem, D. (2020, April 15). Language Learning Apps Are Seeing A Surge In Interest During The COVID-19 Pandemic. NYC, NY. Retrieved August 6, 2020, from https://www.forbes.com/

Center for Behavioral Health Statistics and Quality (CBHSQ). (n.d.). Rockville, MD, USA. Retrieved from https://www.samhsa.gov/data/

Ekeocha, T. C. (2015, April). *The Effecs of Visualization and Guided Imagery in Sports Performance.* Texas State University, San Marcos, Texas. Retrieved August 14, 2020, from Texas State University: https://digital.library.txstate.edu/

Gewoib, S. J. (2015). Working towards successful retirement: older workers and retirees speaking about ageing, change and later life. *Working with Older People, 19*(1), 25-32. Retrieved from https://doi.org/

Jones, D. M. (2011). *The Art of Uncertainty: How to Live in the Mystery of Life and Love It.* NYC, NY, USA: Jeremy P. Tarcher/Penguin. Retrieved from http://dennismerrittjones.com/

Karanen, T. D. (2018, February 1). From the Trailer Park to the Pulpit: Reflections on the wise and wacky sayings of Grandma Esther.

Kofman, Y. B., & Garfin, D. R. (2020, May 8). Home Is Not Always a Haven: The Domestic Violence Crisis Amid the COVID-19 Pandemic. *American Psychological Association: Trauma Psychology*, pp. S199-201.

Kumar, R. (2010). Psychological Preparation for Enhancing the Performance in Sports and Games. *International Journal of*

health, *Physical Education, and Computer Science in Sports,*
37(1). Retrieved August 14 2020, from
https://d1wqtxts1xzle7.cloudfront.net/

Mansfield, A. K., Addis, M. E., & Mahalik, J. R. (2003, May). "Why
Won't He Go to the Doctor?": The Psychology of Men's Help
Seeking. *International Journal of Men's Health, 2*(2), 93-109.

McClure, P. K., & Wilkinson, L. R. (2020, March 13). Attending
Substance Abuse Groups and Identifying as Spiritual but not
Religious. *Review of Religious Research, 62*, pp. 197-218.
Retrieved August 7, 2020, from https://doi.org/

Milner, K. A., Vaccarino, V., Arnold, A. L., Funk, M., & Goldberg, R. J.
(2004). Gender and age differences in chief complaints of
acute myocardial infarction (Worchester heart attack study).
The American Journal of Cardiology, 93(5), 606-608.

Newmark, T. (2012, October 22). Cases in Visualization for Improved
Athletic Performance. *Psychiatric Annals, 42*(10), pp. 385-
387. Retrieved from https://doi.org/

Payne, K., Niemi, L., & Doris, J. (2018, March 27). How to Think About
"Implicit Bias". *Scientific American.* Retrieved from
https://getpocket.com/

Quote Investigator. (2017, November 22). Retrieved August 13,
2020, from https://quoteinvestigator.com/

Schlichthorst, M., Sanci, L. A., Pirlis, J., Spittal, M. J., & Hocking, J. S.
(2016, October 31). Why do men go to the doctor? Socio-
demographic and lifestyle factors associated with healthcare
utilisation among a cohort of Australian men. *BMC Public
Health, 16*, 81-90. Retrieved from https://doi.org/

Shaw, J. (2018). *Pioneers of Modern Spirituality: The Neglected
Anglican Innovators of a "Spiritual but Not Religious" Age.*
London: Darton, Longman and Todd.

Substance Abuse and Mental Health Services Administration
(SAMHSA). (n.d.). Rockville, MD, USA. Retrieved from
https://www.samhsa.gov/

U.S. Department of Health and Human Services (HHS). (n.d.). Washington, DC, USA. Retrieved from https://hhs.gov/

White, R. W., & Horvitz, E. (2009, November 14). Experiences with Web Search on Medical Concerns and Self Diagnosis. *AMIA Annual Symposium Proceedings Archive*, 696-700. Retrieved August 6, 2020, from https://www.ncbi.nlm.nih.gov/

www.ingramcontent.com/pod-product-compliance
Lightning Source LLC
Chambersburg PA
CBHW050533280326
41933CB00011B/1575